# THE ULTIMATE GUIDE TO LOSING 60 POUNDS IN 6 MONTHS: A SIMPLE AND SUSTAINABLE APPROACH

THE ONLY DIET AND EXERCISE PLAN YOU'LL EVER NEED

ESTELLE WOLFE

BETTER YOU ETC. PUBLISHING

Copyright © 2023 by Estelle Wolfe

All rights reserved.

No part of this book may be reproduced in any form or by any electronic or mechanical means, including information storage and retrieval systems, without written permission from the author, except for the use of brief quotations in a book review.

**Disclaimer:**

**\*Be sure to consult with your physician before beginning this program or any program in order to assess your individual needs, tolerance, and abilities.**

# INTRODUCTION

Welcome to "The Ultimate Guide to Losing 60 Pounds in 6 Months: A Simple and Sustainable Approach"! Having gone through the arduous endeavor of losing weight, I understand how tough it is to keep those extra pounds off. With that knowledge in mind, this guide has been formed and aims to assist you on your journey toward a healthier figure.

First, let's talk about why you're here. You want to lose 60 pounds in 6 months, and you're looking for a plan to help you achieve that goal healthily and sustainably. Be assured that losing weight and maintaining the results is a feasible goal, and this guide will provide you with helpful tips and strategies to make it happen.

The first step in any weight loss journey is understanding the basics of weight loss and metabolism. Our bodies are incredibly complex systems, and we must understand how they work to lose weight. To achieve successful weight loss, the key is to burn more calories than we consume. When we eat more calories than our bodies need, the excess is stored as fat. To lose weight, we need to create a calorie deficit by eating less or burning more calories through exercise.

It's also important to understand that weight loss is not just about the number on the scale. It's about improving overall health and fitness. That's why our plan will focus on losing weight and improving nutrition, increasing physical activity, and adopting healthy habits that will benefit you long term.

Now that you have a basic understanding of weight loss and metabolism, it's time to create a personalized plan that works for you. In the next chapter, we will dive deeper into the diet and exercise plan to help you lose 60 pounds in 6 months. But before we do that, I want you to remember that weight loss is a journey, not a destination. It's important to be kind to yourself, set realistic goals and expectations, and remember that progress, not perfection, is the key to success.

I'm excited for you to embark on this journey with me, and I'll be here to guide you every step of the way. Let's get started!

# 1

# SETTING REALISTIC GOALS

Setting goals is essential in any weight loss journey, but it's crucial to ensure they are SMART goals: Specific, Measurable, Achievable, Relevant, and Time-bound.

First, let's talk about being Specific. When setting a weight loss goal, it's essential to be specific about your goal. Instead of saying, "I want to lose weight," try setting a specific goal like "I want to lose 60 pounds in 6 months." Having a specific goal makes it much easier to measure progress and gives you an aim towards which to strive.

Next, make sure your goal is Measurable. You should be able to track your progress and measure your progress. In this case, we'll be measuring your progress in pounds.

Achievable is another critical aspect of a SMART goal. Losing 60 pounds in 6 months is a challenging goal, but it's achievable with the right plan and effort. However, it's important to remember that weight loss differs for everyone, so you may need to adjust your goal based on your circumstances.

The goal should be Relevant to your life; if it's not relevant, it's not worth the effort. It's essential to ensure that your goal is something you genuinely want and will positively impact your life.

Finally, set a Time-bound goal, which means setting a deadline to achieve the goal. A deadline can help you stay focused and motivated, and it also helps you to measure progress.

When setting a weight loss goal, ensure it's Specific, Measurable, Achievable, Relevant, and Time-bound. Losing 60 pounds in 6 months is a challenging goal, but it's achievable with the right plan, effort, and mindset.

# 2

# THE SCIENCE OF WEIGHT LOSS

In this chapter, we're going to dive deeper into the science of weight loss and understand how our bodies work when it comes to weight loss.

As mentioned in Part 1, weight loss is about creating a calorie deficit. A calorie deficit occurs when we burn more calories than we consume. For our bodies to perform optimally, we must take in an adequate number of calories. However, if the caloric intake is higher than what's required for functioning properly, these extra amounts will be stored as fat. To achieve a healthy weight loss journey and create a calorie deficit, it is necessary to eat fewer calories or expend additional energy through physical activity.

But the body is more complex, and weight loss is not just about the number of calories we eat and burn. Our hormones play a significant role in weight loss as well. Hormones like insulin, ghrelin, and leptin regulate our hunger and fullness, and when they're out of balance, weight loss can be more difficult. Understanding how these hormones work and how to balance them is crucial for weight loss success.

Nutrition also plays a vital role in weight loss. Eating a diet high in nutrient-dense foods and low in processed foods can help you lose weight, improve your health, and boost your energy levels. Our diet plan is designed to provide you with the right balance of macronutrients (carbohydrates, proteins, and fats) and micronutrients (vitamins and minerals) to support your weight loss and overall health.

Exercise is also an essential component of weight loss. Regular physical activity burns calories and improves overall health and fitness. Our exercise plan is designed to be personalized, taking into account your fitness level and goals. It's important to find an exercise that you enjoy and that fits into your lifestyle so that you can stick to it.

The science of weight loss is complex and multifaceted. In addition to calorie balance and hormones, several other factors play a role in weight loss, including genetics, metabolism, and lifestyle.

One of the key factors in weight loss is genetics. Our genetics play a role in our body composition, including where we store fat and how our bodies respond to specific diets and exercise. Some people may find it easier to lose weight than others, and this can be due in part to genetics.

Metabolism is another crucial factor in weight loss. Our metabolism is the miraculous process of transforming food into energy, and certain individuals are blessed with a quicker metabolism that assists in weight loss. The speed of your metabolic rate can depend on many factors, such as muscle mass, age, and hormones.

Lifestyle is also a critical factor in weight loss. Factors such as stress, lack of sleep, and sedentary behavior can all contribute to weight gain. Stress can raise cortisol levels, contributing to weight gain, particularly around your abdomen. Lack of sleep can also disrupt hormones that regulate hunger and fullness, making it more difficult to lose weight. On the other hand, sedentary behavior can lead to a decrease in calorie expenditure, making it harder to create a calorie deficit.

Weight loss is a complex process influenced by various factors, including calorie balance, hormones, genetics, metabolism, and lifestyle. To achieve weight loss success, it's essential to take a holistic approach that addresses all of these factors and focuses on making sustainable changes to your diet and lifestyle. This can include making dietary changes, incorporating physical activity, and addressing stress, sleep, and sedentary behavior.

# 3

# THE ROLE OF NUTRITION AND EXERCISE IN WEIGHT LOSS

Nutrition and exercise are two essential components of weight loss. In this section, we will talk about the role of nutrition and exercise in weight loss and how they work together to help you achieve your goals.

First, let's talk about nutrition. The foods we eat provide our bodies with the energy and nutrients they need to function properly. To lose weight, we need to create a calorie deficit, and one of the best ways to do that is by eating a diet that's high in nutrient-dense foods and low in processed foods. Nourishing your body with the right foods - think fruits, vegetables, lean proteins, and healthy fats - can help you shed unwanted pounds and positively affect your overall health and energy levels.

Conversely, excessive consumption of processed items, extra sugars, and saturated fats can result in weight gain and poor well-being. Our diet plan is tailored to offer you a perfect balance of macronutrients (carbohydrates, proteins, and fats) and micronutrients (vitamins and minerals) to keep your weight loss journey on track while improving overall health.

Ready to talk about fitness? Regular exercise not only burns calories but also promotes overall health and wellness! This can help you lose weight by burning fat and building muscle mass; the result is a higher metabolism rate. Additionally, it has been proven that physical activity elevates moods, relieves stress levels, and grants an improved sensation of well-being.

The key to successful weight loss is to find an exercise that you enjoy and that fits into your lifestyle. Our exercise plan is designed to be personalized, taking into account your fitness level and goals. Whether you're new to exercise or an experienced athlete, we have an exercise plan that will work for you.

Nutrition and exercise are both important components of weight loss. Eating a healthy diet that's high in nutrient-dense foods and low in processed foods while, at the same time, engaging in regular physical activity can help you lose weight, improve your health, and boost your energy levels.

# 4

# COMMON WEIGHT LOSS MYTHS

You've likely heard all kinds of gossip about weight loss--from fad diets and pills that are said to be "miracle cures" to the latest trends. But what's real and what's not? We'll explore some of the most common myths surrounding shedding pounds, so you can get informed on which theories hold.

MYTH 1: Crash diets and extreme calorie restriction are the best way to lose weight. Crash diets and extreme calorie restrictions may result in weight loss in the short term, but they are not sustainable in the long term. Crash diets can lead to nutrient deficiencies, muscle loss, and a slowed metabolism. Additionally, they can also lead to binge eating, and weight regain. It's important to remember that weight loss is a journey, not a destination, and sustainable weight loss comes from making small, gradual changes to your diet and lifestyle.

MYTH 2: Eating fat makes you fat. Eating fat does not make you fat. Healthy fats like those found in avocado, nuts, and seeds are important for maintaining good health and feeling full. Not all fats are created equal, and it's important to focus on eating healthy fats and limiting saturated and trans fats.

**MYTH 3:** Carbs are the enemy. To stay healthy and feel your best, it is essential to prioritize complex carbohydrates from sources like fruits, vegetables, and whole grains. Simultaneously be mindful of limiting the intake of simple carbs such as white bread or sugary beverages to sustain good health. After all, carbohydrates are an essential energy source for our bodies!

**MYTH 4:** You can target specific body areas for weight loss. Targeting specific areas of your body for weight loss is impossible. Your body loses weight in a specific order, and your genetics determines it. You can't change where your body loses weight first, but you can change your overall body composition by losing fat and gaining muscle through a healthy diet and regular exercise.

**MYTH 5:** Skipping meals will help you lose weight. Skipping meals can be counter-productive for weight loss. Skipping meals can cause your body to enter "starvation mode" and slow down your metabolism. Additionally, skipping meals can lead to overeating later in the day and disrupt blood sugar levels. Instead of skipping meals, try to eat small, regular meals throughout the day to keep your metabolism running and your blood sugar levels stable.

**MYTH 6:** Weight loss supplements and detox teas are the keys to weight loss success. Weight loss supplements and detox teas are not the magic solution to weight loss. Many of these products lack scientific evidence to support their claims and can even harm your health. Additionally, weight loss supplements and detox teas do not address the root causes of weight gain and are not a sustainable solution. A healthy diet and regular exercise is the best way to lose weight and keep it off.

**MYTH 7:** You have to exercise for hours daily to see results. It's okay to exercise for hours a day to see results. Even small amounts of exercise can have a significant impact on weight loss. Research shows that moderate-intensity exercise, such as a brisk walk, for 30 minutes daily, can help you lose weight and improve your overall health. The key is to find an exercise that you enjoy and that fits into your lifestyle so that you can stick to it.

Weight loss is a complex process, and there is a lot of misinformation. Remember to be skeptical of quick-fix solutions and focus on making small, gradual changes to your diet and lifestyle.

5
---

# THE DIET PLAN

This dietary plan helps you achieve your weight-loss goals and encourages complete physical and mental health. This system is founded on the concept of calorie deficit – meaning that consumption will be less than expenditure.

Starting with macronutrients, Carbohydrates are an essential part of the diet, providing the body with energy. The plan includes complex carbohydrates such as whole grains, fruits, and vegetables, which are high in fiber and nutrients and can help to keep you feeling full for longer. These types of carbohydrates are also rich in vitamins and minerals and are a great energy source. To avoid a rise in blood sugar and excess weight gain, limit your consumption of simple carbohydrates like white bread, sugar, and sugary drinks.

Proteins are also a crucial part of the diet. They are important for building and repairing muscle. The plan includes lean proteins such as chicken, fish, and tofu and plant-based proteins like beans and lentils. These protein sources are also nutrient-dense and provide essential amino acids necessary for maintaining muscle mass and preventing muscle loss.

Healthy fats are also included in the plan. Replenishing your diet with healthy fats, such as avocado, nuts, seeds, and olive oil, can be critical for attaining maximum wellness. They also help absorb specific vitamins and minerals that can otherwise be difficult to get from other sources. While including them in your diet is beneficial, it's important not to overdo it on saturated or trans fats - these have been linked to higher risks of heart disease.

Micronutrients, including vitamins and minerals, are also essential in the diet and are found in fruits, vegetables, and whole grains. The plan includes various fruits and vegetables to provide the necessary vitamins and minerals. With relatively few calories and high fiber content, these foods are the perfect option for aiding in weight loss.

The diet plan is crafted to be adaptive and personalizable to ensure that you can successfully and sustainably attain your desired results. It's essential to find a balance that works for you in the long run; consequently, it'd be beneficial to seek advice from either a healthcare professional or a certified nutritionist who can develop an individualized scheme explicitly tailored to your particular needs and objectives.

**Meal Plan Examples and Recipes**

**Day 1:**
Breakfast: Whole grain toast laden with creamy avocado and a poached egg.

- To make this meal, toast two slices of whole-grain bread. While the bread is toasting, mash half an avocado and spread it on the toast. Then, poach one egg and place it on top of the avocado toast.

Snack: Greek yogurt with berries

- To make this snack, take a cup of Greek yogurt and mix it with a handful of mixed berries. You can also add some honey or a sprinkle of cinnamon for added flavor.

Lunch: Savory grilled chicken breast alongside hearty quinoa and succulent steamed vegetables.

- To make this meal, grill a chicken breast and season it with your favorite herbs and spices. Cook a cup of quinoa according to package instructions. Steam a cup of your favorite vegetables, such as broccoli, bell peppers, and carrots. Serve the chicken breast on top of the quinoa and vegetables.

Snack: Apple slices with almond butter

- To make this snack, slice an apple and spread a tablespoon of almond butter. You can also add a sprinkle of cinnamon for added flavor.

Dinner: Oven-roasted salmon, accompanied by the perfect side dish of sweet potato and green beans.

- To make this meal, preheat the oven to 375 degrees F. Place a salmon fillet on a baking sheet lined with parchment paper. Bake for 12-15 minutes or until cooked through. Cut a sweet potato into wedges and toss with olive oil, salt, and pepper. Roast in the oven for 20-25 minutes. Steam a cup of green beans for 5-7 minutes. Serve the salmon with sweet potato wedges and green beans.

Day 2:
Breakfast: Ultimate overnight oats- chia seeds, berries, and your favorite fixings!

- To make this meal, mix 1/2 cup of rolled oats, 1/2 cup of milk, 1/2 cup of Greek yogurt, one tablespoon of chia seeds, and a handful of mixed berries in a jar or container. Cover and refrigerate overnight. Add a little bit of honey or maple syrup in the morning for added sweetness, and enjoy!

Snack: Veggie and hummus wrap

- To make this snack, spread hummus on a whole wheat wrap and add your favorite vegetables, such as cucumber, tomato, bell pepper, and lettuce. Roll it up and enjoy!

Lunch: Turkey and veggie stir-fry

- To make this meal, cook a cup of brown rice according to the package instructions. In a separate pan, heat a tablespoon of olive oil. Stir-fried sliced turkey and vegetables such as bell peppers, broccoli, and carrots. Season with your favorite stir-fry sauce and serve over the brown rice.

Snack: Celery sticks with peanut butter

- To make this snack, cut celery into sticks and spread a teaspoon of peanut butter on each one. You can also add raisins for added sweetness.

Dinner: Baked chicken breast with roasted vegetables

- To make this meal, preheat the oven to 375 degrees F. Place a chicken breast on a baking sheet lined with parchment paper. Bake for 20-25 minutes. Cut vegetables such as bell peppers, broccoli, and cauliflower into bite-size pieces and toss with olive oil, salt, and pepper. Roast in the oven for 20-25 minutes. Serve the chicken breast with roasted vegetables.

**Day 3:**
Breakfast: Egg and vegetable scramble

- Heat a tablespoon of olive oil over medium heat to make this meal. Add your favorite veggies, such as bell peppers, onions, mushrooms, and spinach. Cook until softened. Beat two eggs in a small bowl, add them to the pan, and scramble until cooked—season with salt and pepper to taste. Serve with whole-grain toast.

Snack: Cottage cheese and fruit salad

- To make this snack, mix 1 cup of cottage cheese with your favorite fruits such as berries, apples, and peaches. Add a sprinkle of cinnamon or a drizzle of honey for added flavor.

Lunch: Tuna salad lettuce wraps

- To make this meal, mix a can of drained and flaked tuna with a tablespoon of mayonnaise, diced celery, a diced onion, and a tablespoon of lemon juice—season with salt and pepper to taste. Serve the tuna salad in lettuce leaves.

Snack: Baked sweet potato wedges

- To make this snack, preheat the oven to 400 degrees F. Cut a sweet potato into wedges and toss with olive oil, salt, and pepper. Roast in the oven for 20-25 minutes.

Dinner: Grilled shrimp and zucchini pasta

- To make this meal, cook a cup of whole wheat pasta according to package instructions. Heat a tablespoon of olive oil separately and grill shrimp and zucchini until cooked. Toss the pasta with the shrimp and zucchini, and season with your favorite pasta sauce.

**Day 4:**
Breakfast: Berry and quinoa bowl

- To make this meal, cook a cup of quinoa according to the package instructions. Once it's cooked, mix it with a cup of mixed berries and a drizzle of honey. Top with a spoonful of Greek yogurt and a sprinkle of chopped nuts.

Snack: Carrot sticks and hummus

- To make this snack, cut carrots into sticks and serve with a side of hummus for dipping.

Lunch: Turkey and avocado lettuce wraps

- To make this meal, mix sliced turkey, diced avocado, tomatoes, and red onion—season with salt, pepper, and lemon juice. Serve the mixture in lettuce leaves.

Snack: Cucumber and feta cheese

- To make this snack, slice cucumber and top with crumbled feta cheese and a sprinkle of dill.

Dinner: Oven roasted Cod with a side of roasted vegetables

- To make this meal, preheat the oven to 375 degrees F. Place a cod fillet on a baking sheet lined with parchment paper. Bake for 12-15 minutes or until cooked through. Cut vegetables such as bell peppers, broccoli, and cauliflower into bite-size pieces and toss with olive oil, salt, and pepper. Roast in the oven for 20-25 minutes. Serve the cod fillet with the roasted vegetables.

### Day 5:

Breakfast: Veggie and turkey bacon omelet

- To make this meal, beat two eggs in a bowl and season with salt and pepper. Heat a non-stick skillet over medium heat and add diced vegetables such as bell peppers, onion, mushrooms, and spinach. Cook until softened. Add two strips of turkey bacon and cook until crispy. Pour the eggs over the vegetables and turkey bacon and scramble until cooked.

Snack: Banana and almond butter

- To make this snack, slice a banana and spread a tablespoon of almond butter.

Lunch: Grilled chicken Caesar salad

- To make this meal, grill a chicken breast and slice it into strips. Toss the chicken with romaine lettuce, croutons, and a classic Caesar dressing.

Snack: hard-boiled eggs

- To make this snack, place eggs in a saucepan and cover with cold water. Bring water to a boil, then cover and remove from heat. Let eggs stand in hot water for 12 to 15 minutes. Drain and cool the eggs under cold running water, peel the eggs and enjoy

Dinner: Slow-cooker beef and vegetable stew

- To make this meal, add a pound of beef stew meat, diced potatoes, carrots, and onions to a slow cooker. Add beef broth, tomato paste, and your favorite seasonings. Cook on low for 8 hours.

These recipes are easy to make and packed with nutrients. These meals can help you to achieve your weight loss goals while keeping you healthy and satisfied. Remember, to make it more effective, it's recommended to consult a healthcare professional or a registered dietitian who can help you to create a more personalized meal plan that addresses your unique needs and goals.

## 6

# TIPS FOR GROCERY SHOPPING AND MEAL PREP

Grocery shopping and meal prep are essential aspects of any weight loss journey. By planning ahead and making smart choices at the grocery store, you can set yourself up for success and make sticking to your diet plan much easier.

When stocking up on supplies, it's critical to plan ahead and stay committed to that list. This will prevent unnecessary impulse buys and assist in maintaining your diet goals. Compose a menu of nutrient-rich produce, lean proteins, and whole grains – they'll keep hunger at bay while providing essential nutrients. Steer clear of processed snacks; they typically contain too many calories without supplying the much-needed nutrition!

Another tip for grocery shopping is to shop the perimeter of the store. This is where you'll find fresh produce, meats, and dairy products, whereas processed foods are typically found in the middle aisles. By focusing on the store's perimeter, you'll be more likely to make healthy choices.

Regarding meal prep, it's important to set aside time each week to plan your meals and prepare ingredients. This can include washing and cutting fruits and vegetables, cooking grains, and prepping proteins. Meal prepping also allows you to make large batches of food that can be portioned and eaten throughout the week, saving you time and energy.

Another excellent way to streamline your meal planning is to use leftovers. Think outside the box and cook an extra portion of dinner or lunch one day so you can enjoy it the next! Not only will this save you time and energy, but it will also cut down on food wastage.

If there's ever a week that requires quick solutions, don't be afraid to take advantage of pre-prepared ingredients or opt for meals that require minimal effort and time investment — with no sacrifice in taste! Be flexible yet practical about how much effort goes into your weekly meal prep process.

Another tip for meal prep is to make use of your freezer. You can make large batches of food, such as soups, stews, and casseroles, and freeze them in individual portions. This way, you always have a healthy meal ready to go when you don't have time to cook.

Regarding grocery shopping, it's also important to be mindful of the ingredients in the products you buy. Read the labels, look for items with fewer ingredients, and avoid items containing added sugars and artificial ingredients.

Another important aspect of grocery shopping is awareness of the products' cost. Try to stick to your budget and look for deals and sales on products that you regularly use. Also, consider buying bulk items that have a long shelf life, such as rice, beans, and oats, as it can save you money in the long run.

Finally, consider incorporating more plant-based options into your diet. By incorporating an abundance of plant-based foods such as fruits, vegetables, whole grains, and legumes into your diet plan, you can benefit from their high fiber and nutrient content that is low in calories - a perfect combination to aid weight loss!

Grocery shopping and meal prep are essential aspects of any weight loss journey. By planning, making intelligent choices at the grocery store, being mindful of the ingredients, being aware of the cost, and incorporating more plant-based options into your diet, you can set yourself up for success and make sticking to your diet plan much easier.

# 7
# THE EXERCISE PLAN

Exercise is vital in any weight loss regimen, as it burns calories and boosts overall fitness and well-being. To make the most out of your exercise routine, you should include an equal share of cardio workouts, strength exercises, and flexibility/mobility drills for optimal results.

**Cardiovascular exercise**, more commonly known as cardio, is an activity that quickens your pulse and circulates blood throughout the body. Popular types of cardio include walking, running, biking, swimming, or dancing. According to The American College of Sports Medicine's guidelines for adults: you should be doing at least 150 minutes a week of moderate-intensity cardio or 75 minutes a week (if it's vigorous-intensity). So don't wait any longer - get those heart rates soaring!

**Resistance training**, or strength training as it's more commonly known, is any exercise that requires your muscles to exert effort. This can include weightlifting, bodyweight exercises, and resistance band workouts. It is recommended that adults engage in a minimum of two days of strength training per week for optimal health benefits.

**Flexibility and mobility exercises**, also known as stretching, help to improve the range of motion in the joints and muscles. Examples of flexibility and mobility exercises include yoga, Pilates, and stretching. At least two days of flexibility and mobility exercises per week for adults are recommended.

It's important to note that the frequency and intensity of exercise will depend on your individual fitness level and goals. Consult a healthcare professional or a certified personal trainer to help create a personalized exercise plan that addresses your unique needs and goals.

In addition to the recommended types of exercise, it's also important to focus on proper form and technique to prevent injury and ensure maximum results. It's also important to listen to your body and adjust if you're feeling overly tired or experiencing pain; rest and recover before continuing.

A well-rounded exercise plan that combines cardiovascular exercise, strength training, and flexibility/mobility exercises is essential for weight loss and overall health and well-being. However, it's important to remember that the frequency and intensity of exercise will depend on your individual fitness level and goals. Consult a healthcare professional or a certified personal trainer to help create a personalized exercise plan that addresses your unique needs and goals.

It's also important to focus on proper form and technique to prevent injury and ensure maximum results. Make sure to listen to your body and adjust if you're feeling overly tired or experiencing pain; rest and recover before continuing.

It's also important to remember that weight loss is not only about calories burned during exercise but also about the number of calories consumed. Therefore, it's essential to have a well-balanced diet that supports your weight loss goals. Exercise should be combined with a healthy and balanced diet for optimal results.

Finally, finding an exercise you enjoy and can stick to is important. This will make it easier to maintain an active lifestyle and more enjoyable. You can try different types of exercise to find what you enjoy most and what fits into your schedule. This will help to make exercise a sustainable and long-term lifestyle change that can help you to achieve your weight loss goals.

*For more workouts that are at a beginner level and beyond. I highly recommend this Youtube channel. It's awesome!!

# 8

# DESIGNING A WORKOUT SCHEDULE

Crafting an exercise regime that works for you can be difficult, but reaching your desired weight loss outcomes is necessary. The trick lies in finding the right mix of reliability and adaptability; make sure your workout program complements your daily routine. With a tailored schedule, hitting those targets will become much more attainable!

First, it's important to set realistic goals for yourself. If you're new to exercise, start with small, manageable goals and work your way up. For example, start with just a few minutes of exercise a day and gradually increase the duration and intensity over time.

Next, find a time of day that works best for you to exercise. Some people prefer to exercise in the morning, while others prefer to exercise in the evening. Experiment with different times of the day to find what works best for you.

In addition, it's essential to be flexible with your workout schedule. Life can be unpredictable, and it's crucial to be able to adjust your workout schedule as needed. For example, if you have a busy day at work, you might need to adjust your workout schedule to accommodate it.

Another important aspect is finding an exercise you enjoy and can stick to. This will make it easier to maintain an active lifestyle and more enjoyable. You can try different types of exercise to find what you enjoy most and what fits into your schedule. This will help to make exercise a sustainable and long-term lifestyle change that can help you to achieve your weight loss goals.

Lastly, it's important to remember that consistency is key. You don't have to exercise for hours every day to see results. Even just a few minutes of exercise a day can make a difference. The most important thing is to make exercise a regular part of your life and stick to it.

Remember to start with small, manageable goals, find a time of day that works best for you, be flexible and find an exercise you enjoy and can maintain.

# 9

## COMMON EXERCISE OBSTACLES AND HOW TO OVERCOME THEM

When it comes to exercise, it's normal to encounter obstacles and challenges. However, recognizing and addressing these obstacles, you can overcome them and stay on track with your weight loss goals.

One common obstacle is the need for more time. Many people need help to fit exercise into their busy schedules. One solution to this problem is to schedule exercises like any other necessary appointment. Carve out a few days each week to exercise and make it an absolute must, or try fitting physical activity into your daily life, such as taking the stairs rather than an elevator; you can also opt for walking or cycling instead of driving to work.

Another common obstacle is a need for more motivation. It's easy to lose motivation when you don't see immediate results or progress seems slow. To overcome this obstacle, try to focus on the benefits of exercise beyond weight loss, such as improved mood, better sleep, and increased energy levels. Also, set small, attainable goals and reward yourself when you reach them.

Lack of variety in your exercise routine can also be an obstacle, leading to boredom and lack of interest. To overcome this obstacle, try new activities, such as hiking, swimming, or dancing, or switch up your gym routine by incorporating new exercises or equipment. Joining a fitness class or working out with a friend can add variety and make exercise more enjoyable.

Injury is another obstacle preventing you from continuing your exercise routine. To prevent injury:

1. Warm up properly before exercising and cool down afterward.
2. Use proper form and technique, and don't push yourself too hard too quickly.
3. If you experience an injury, consult a healthcare professional and follow their recommendations for recovery and rehabilitation.

Finally, lack of support can also be an obstacle, as it can be challenging to stick to an exercise routine without the encouragement and support of others. To overcome this obstacle, find a workout buddy or join a fitness community to share your progress and get motivation and encouragement.

These common exercise obstacles, such as lack of time, lack of motivation, lack of variety in your exercise routine, injury, and lack of support, can make it challenging to stick to your weight loss goals. However, by recognizing and addressing these obstacles, you can overcome them and stay on track.

# 10

# THE IMPORTANCE OF A POSITIVE MINDSET

Regarding weight loss, it's easy to focus on the numbers on the scale and the inches we want to lose. However, it's essential to remember that weight loss is not only about physical changes but also mental and emotional changes. A positive mindset is crucial in weight loss, as it can help keep you motivated, focused, and on track.

To begin with, a positive outlook will help you remain in the moment and appreciate your weight loss effort. Rather than put all of your energy into achieving a result, try to savor the small but significant transformations you'll observe throughout this process - physical or mental changes. Remember: Losing weight is a journey, not just a destination, so enjoy every step along the way!

A positive mindset can also help you to stay motivated and focused. When you're feeling down or discouraged, it can be easy to fall off track and give up on your goals. However, with a positive mindset, you can remind yourself of why you started and your progress, which can keep you motivated and focused on your goals.

A positive mindset can also help you stay consistent with your diet and exercise plan. When you're in a positive state of mind, you're more likely to make healthy choices and stick to your plan. On the other hand, when you're feeling down or discouraged, it can be easy to fall into bad habits and give up on your goals.

Finally, having a positive attitude can help you develop an encouraging relationship with food and exercise. Rather than treating them like rules or punishments, recognize that they are assets to assist you in reaching your objectives and advancing your health. With the right mindset, these activities will no longer feel overwhelming but become enjoyable habits that contribute to both physical and mental well-being.

Having a positive mindset is crucial when it comes to weight loss. It can help you to focus on the present moment and enjoy the journey, stay motivated and focused, stay consistent and develop a healthy relationship with food and exercise. Remember, weight loss is not only about physical, mental, and emotional changes. By adopting a positive mindset, you'll be able to achieve your goals and improve your overall health and well-being.

# 11

# STRATEGIES FOR STAYING MOTIVATED AND OVERCOMING SETBACKS

Staying motivated and overcoming setbacks are essential parts of any weight loss journey. However, it's normal to encounter obstacles and challenges along the way. The key is to have strategies to help you stay motivated and overcome setbacks when they happen.

One strategy for staying motivated is setting small, attainable goals. Instead of focusing on the result, focus on the small, positive changes in your body and mind. When you reach a goal, reward yourself, it can be something small like buying a new book or going out for a nice dinner. Setting small goals will help you to stay motivated and focused on your journey.

Another strategy for staying motivated is to surround yourself with positive influences. This can include friends, family members, or a supportive community that can offer encouragement and support. Joining a support group or working with a personal trainer can also be helpful.

To overcome setbacks, it's important to have a plan in place. This can include identifying triggers that lead to setbacks and developing strategies to avoid them. For example, if you know that stress or boredom leads you to overeat, you can develop a plan to address these triggers, such as going for a walk or calling a friend when you feel stressed.

It's also important to be kind to yourself and practice self-compassion. Setbacks are a normal part of any journey, and it's important to remember that it's not about perfection but progress. Be kind to yourself and remember that it's okay to slip up and make mistakes.

Finally, it's essential to focus on the bigger picture. Remember why you started your weight loss journey and focus on the benefits that come with it, such as improved health, more energy, and better overall well-being. Keeping the bigger picture in mind will help you to stay motivated and overcome setbacks.

Keeping motivated and rising above obstacles are two essential steps in any weight loss journey. To stay inspired, set achievable goals for yourself, engage with encouraging people around you, and establish a well-thought action plan.

# 12

# BUILDING A SUPPORT SYSTEM

Establishing a support system is essential for successful weight loss. With it, you can remain motivated, concentrated, and aligned with your objectives. Additionally, having assistance in place will permit you to confront roadblocks when they arise. To assemble a dependable system of help, reach out to those closest to you - friends and family members - by sharing your intentions with them and explaining how they can be there for you whenever needed – whether as an exercise companion or someone willing to chat during times of discouragement!

Another way to build a support system is to join a weight loss group or community. These groups can provide you with a sense of belonging and camaraderie, and you can share your progress and challenges with others who are going through the same thing. Many online communities, weight loss groups, and forums can be great ways to connect with like-minded people who are also on a weight loss journey.

Working with a personal trainer or a dietitian can also be a great way to build a support system. A personal trainer can help you develop a personalized workout plan that addresses your unique needs and goals and provides motivation, accountability, and guidance. A dietitian can help you to develop a healthy and balanced diet plan that supports your weight loss goals.

It's also important to build a support system for yourself. This can include journaling, meditation, or yoga to help you stay focused and motivated. Self-care activities such as reading, listening to music, or walking can also be helpful.

Forming a support network is essential to achieving your weight loss objectives. With the right encouragement and reinforcement, you can remain motivated while keeping yourself on track toward successful results. Reach out to friends and family members, join a weight loss group or community, work with a personal trainer or dietitian, and build a support system for yourself. Remember that you don't have to go through this process alone. A strong support system can make all the difference when reaching your desired weight loss goals.

# 13

# LONG-TERM WEIGHT LOSS MAINTENANCE

Congratulations on completing your 6-month weight loss plan! This is a significant achievement, and you should be proud of yourself for all the hard work and dedication you've put in. But now, the question is, what's next? How do you transition from the 6-month plan to long-term weight maintenance?

First and foremost, it's important to remember that weight maintenance is a continuous process. It's not a destination but a journey. The key is to make healthy habits a part of your daily routine rather than a temporary fix.

One of the best ways to transition to long-term weight maintenance is to continue following a healthy diet and exercise plan. This doesn't mean that you have to be strict and restrictive all the time, but it's important to find a balance that works for you. You can continue to use the principles of the diet plan you followed during the 6-month plan, but allow yourself some flexibility to enjoy your favorite foods in moderation. The same goes for exercise; continue to find an activity you enjoy and make it a part of your routine.

It's also important to continue to set goals for yourself. These goals can be related to weight loss, fitness, or overall health. Having a goal to work towards helps keep you motivated and focused.

Another important aspect of transitioning to long-term weight maintenance is to develop a healthy relationship with food and exercise. Instead of viewing them as restrictions or punishments, view them as tools to help you achieve your goals and improve your overall health and well-being.

Finally, it's essential to continue to build a support system. Reach out to friends and family members, join a weight loss group or community, work with a personal trainer or dietitian, and build a support system for yourself. Don't forget; you don't have to go through this alone. A support network around you makes achieving your weight loss goals all the more achievable.

Ultimately, transitioning from a 6-month plan to sustained weight maintenance is a continuous process. To be successful, you must adhere to a healthy diet and exercise routines; establish objectives for yourself; build healthier relationships with food and physical activity; and focus on growing your support system. Weight management should not just be viewed as an endpoint but instead seen as part of the lifelong journey ahead of you. With commitment and flexibility in adjusting when required, victory can surely be yours!

# 14

# TIPS FOR STAYING ON TRACK AND AVOIDING WEIGHT REGAIN

Staying on track and avoiding weight regain can be challenging, but it is an essential part of any weight loss journey. The key is to have strategies in place to help you stay motivated and on track and to be mindful of the potential obstacles that can lead to weight regain.

Finding a balance between health-promoting nutrition and pleasurable indulgences is key to success. Don't feel pressured to be overly restrictive or hard on yourself; instead, stay true to the principles of the 6-month plan you followed while allowing some room for flexibility so that you can still enjoy your favorite foods in moderation. Additionally, make exercise enjoyable by participating in activities that motivate and inspire you; this will become part of your routine!

Another important tip for staying on track is having a plan for dealing with setbacks and challenges. This can include identifying triggers that lead to setbacks, such as stress or boredom, and developing strategies to avoid them. For example, if you know that stress leads you to overeat, you can develop a plan to address this trigger, such as going for a walk or calling a friend when you feel stressed.

It's also important to be mindful of the scale and focus on the numbers. Instead of fixating on the scale, focus on the other positive changes in your body and mind, such as improved energy levels and better sleep.

Additionally, it's important to continue to set goals for yourself. These goals can be related to weight loss, fitness, or overall health. Having a goal to work towards helps keep you motivated and focused.

Another important aspect of avoiding weight regain is to develop a healthy relationship with food and exercise. Instead of viewing them as restrictions or punishments, view them as tools to help you achieve your goals and improve your overall health and well-being.

Finally, it's essential to continue to build a support system. Reach out to friends and family members, join a weight loss group or community, work with a personal trainer or dietitian, and build a support system for yourself. Remember, you are not alone on this journey, and having a support system can make all the difference in achieving your weight loss goals.

# 15

# THE IMPORTANCE OF SELF-CARE AND OVERALL WELL-BEING

Regarding weight loss, it's easy to focus on the numbers on the scale and the inches we want to lose. However, it's essential to remember that weight loss is not only about physical changes but also mental and emotional changes. This is where self-care and overall well-being come into play.

Self-care is taking care of your physical, mental, and emotional well-being. It's about ensuring that you're taking care of yourself physically and mentally to be the best version of yourself. When you take care of yourself, you'll be better equipped to care for others and achieve your weight loss goals.

Achieving adequate rest is one of the essential elements of self-care. Sleep isn't just vital for our physical and mental health. It's also necessary if you're trying to shed some pounds. When we don't get enough sleep, our hormones become imbalanced in a way that increases hunger - ghrelin is released, which stimulates appetite. At the same time, leptin production decreases, leading to more significant cravings. To keep your waistline trim and body healthy, prioritize getting ample shut-eye each night!

Stress management is an integral part of self-care. Unchecked stress can lead to overeating and weight gain and hurt our mental health. Fortunately, there are many ways we can manage our stress levels; find activities we enjoy, such as reading, listening to music, or going for a walk. Ensure these activities become daily rituals in your life!

Taking the time to indulge in what you enjoy is essential to self-care. A bubble bath, reading a novel, or taking a stroll are great ways to do this. It's important to prioritize your own happiness by making time for yourself. Meditation, yoga, or journaling can help replenish energy levels while reducing stress and generating clarity of thought - ultimately contributing to overall well-being!

It's also essential to ensure you get regular check-ups with your healthcare provider to ensure that your overall health is on track. This includes regular screenings, such as blood pressure, cholesterol, and blood sugar, and any other tests or screenings that your healthcare provider recommends.

Self-care and overall well-being are crucial when it comes to weight loss. By incorporating self-care practices, such as getting enough sleep, managing stress, making time for yourself, and focusing on overall well-being, you'll be better equipped to achieve your weight loss goals and improve your overall health and well-being.

## 16

## CLOSING THOUGHTS AND MOTIVATION FOR THE FUTURE

Congratulations on completing this book on how to lose 60 pounds in 6 months! This journey has been filled with challenges and triumphs, but you've made it to the end. Now, it's time to look forward to the future and the opportunities ahead.

As you look to the future, remember that weight loss is a continuous process. It's not a destination but a journey. The key is to make healthy habits a part of your daily routine rather than a temporary fix.

To maintain your progress going forward, it's crucial to adhere to a nutritious diet and exercise routine. You don't have to always be restrictive but find balance. Utilize the principles of the program you followed during these 6 months as a guide, yet allow yourself some flexibility for the occasional indulgence. With physical activity, keep having fun by finding an enjoyable workout that becomes part of your daily schedule so that lasting results are achievable!

It's also important to continue to set goals for yourself. These goals can be related to weight loss, fitness, or overall health. Having a goal to work towards helps keep you motivated and focused.

Another critical aspect of avoiding weight regain is to develop a healthy relationship with food and exercise. Instead of viewing them as restrictions or punishments, view them as tools to help you achieve your goals and improve your overall health and well-being.

Finally, it's essential to continue to build a support system. Reach out to friends and family members, join a weight loss group or community, work with a personal trainer or dietitian, and build a support system for yourself. Remember, you are not alone on this journey, and having a support system can make all the difference in achieving your weight loss goals.

As you move forward, remember that weight loss is not a one-time event, it's a lifestyle change. It's about making healthy choices that support your weight loss goals and being kind and compassionate to yourself.

Remember, you got this! You've made it this far, and with determination and willingness to adapt, you can continue to achieve your weight loss goals in the future.

# 17

# ADDITIONAL RESOURCES FOR FAST TRACK

Here are a couple of products if you are looking to fast-track your results.

Be sure to consult with your physician before you start this program or any program or consume any supplements.

All the best:)

LEAN BELLY SUPPLEMENT

ULTIMATE KETO PLAN

Printed in Great Britain
by Amazon